MOTH TO FLAME

An offline method for new & old PTs to rapidly pick up new clients.

How I built my client base from £0.00 to £2,000.00 in just 9 weeks.

Without social media.

AN OFFLINE LEAD GENERATION PROTOCOL FOR NEW PERSONAL TRAINERS

MOTH TO FLAME

AN OFFLINE LEAD GENERATION PROTOCOL FOR NEW PERSONAL TRAINERS

By:

Emmanuel Salami BSc

CONTENTS

MOTH TO FLAME

AN OFFLINE LEAD GENERATION PROTOCOL FOR NEW PERSONAL TRAINERS

PREFACE

So, you've finished your PT course, got yourself into a gym, excited to start your new career but then NOTHING! You became a personal trainer to train people, but you don't have anyone to train.

Just like I did, you realized your first major task is getting the clients to train in the first place.

At that point, I started reading books and doing research about anything that could help with this initial hurdle, I tried a bunch of things with varying levels of success, some of which I will talk about in the later stages of this book.

After about 3 years of trial and error, there is one thing I started doing that helped me to rapidly gain clients more than anything else, this one thing I have labelled the "Moth to Flame" protocol.

The more I used this protocol for picking up new clients the more I improved upon it and made small nuance tweaks to the process of implementing the protocol. These small changes increased its success and conversion rate even more.

These small changes in my process were not something a book could have told me, they came about through my own trial and error and lived experience of seeing what worked, what got a better reaction from people, and I made those changes as I went along.

When I moved to another gym with zero client base, I didn't waste time with any of the techniques I had learned or tried in the years previous. I went straight into executing my "Moth to Flame" protocol and built up a client base from £0 to £2,000 monthly income in just 9 weeks!

Why stop at £2,000? In my case my 1-2-1 availability at the time was limited, I was working 3 hours an evening 5 days a week, and had no availability for more, I will go into the details of this later in the book.

As a PT with more time, you can use this approach to build up your earnings to £4,000 per month and above, it's a rinse-and-repeat process.

In this book, I will be going into the details of this offline protocol to help you as a new or existing personal trainer, so that you can do the same and save yourself 3 years of experimenting!

I will go into details of how an offline protocol such as the "Moth to Flame" can put you in the driver's seat and help you to feel more in control of your business.

MOTH TO FLAME

AN OFFLINE LEAD GENERATION PROTOCOL FOR NEW PERSONAL TRAINERS

ABOUT THIS BOOK

When you start doing research into how to build a successful personal training business, you will hear over and over again that you need to "master sales skills". This is 100% true, but that's usually where the advice ends. What exactly does selling look like? What exactly do you need to do?

In this book, I will be going into detail about the exact, easy-to-replicate lead generation technique that has worked for me.

We live in a social media age; however, I was never a massive user of social media and I have worked with many personal trainers who aren't either, but you feel like it's something you have to do if you want to see success as a personal trainer in this day and age. The protocol discussed in this book is one way you can see success as a personal trainer without a big social media following.

As the saying goes, "There are many ways to skin a cat". When it comes to personal training, the use of social media is one of them, however, it is only really effective if you have an engaged audience of a decent size and are willing to commit to keeping that audience engaged. In my own judgment, it is also a passive and unpredictable approach to picking up new clients.

Moth to Flame is an offline and proactive method of picking up clients that puts you in the driver's seat with more control of your own destiny. It worked for me, and the same exact protocol can work for you too.

I will detail the approach I took to help me build up my client base in just 9 weeks, down to the details of the exact script I used when speaking with potential clients, including my exact opening phrases and responses to potential clients.

I give detailed examples of other methods I have tried in the past and discuss why they were not as effective as the "Moth to Flame" protocol.

Having a good strategy is one thing, successfully executing it is another. That's why in this book I will also discuss the most important factor that will influence your success in implementing this protocol and the different things you can do to get that one thing working in your favour.

This is an approach that can be used to build your business up to whatever level you want and build up your sessions to whatever your availability allows.

For me at the time, at around £2,000 per month, my availability was fully booked. However, depending on your aspirations and availability, you can use the same exact protocol to earn as much as you want.

Research has shown that around 80% of personal trainers fail within the first year, going into your first year with this protocol will put you miles ahead of the curve.

All the information discussed in this book is from lived experience and my own trial and error. I have read around the internet, read books, tried a whole bunch of things, and developed a method that works, it's a combination of things I have learned from everything I've researched, the influences of other people, and my own personal experience and flair.

This book is not in any way against the use of social media or preaching against using social media. Social media is a great tool to use, however for reasons that are personal to me (which I will discuss in the about me section of this book) I was not great at it and therefore had to adapt to gain clients in other ways, it turns out many other personal trainers also were not massive fans of the use of social media but felt like they had to use it or didn't feel in control of their business.

If you can use social media to your advantage, you definitely should. However, if you are not the type to post a lot on social media or just not that way inclined, this book hopes to reveal that you can 100% be a very successful personal trainer whilst doing your lead generation offline.

Who is this book for?

If you are going to successfully implement the strategy in this book, you will need a good pool of potential clients.

So, this book is for a personal trainer who works in a commercial gym or an aspiring personal trainer who plans on working in commercial gyms.

Commercial gyms typically have high foot traffic and a high number of gym members who are all your potential clients, the people in commercial gyms are a better target audience than any Instagram page where a large portion of the followers can be people who have no interest in your personal training services and maybe not even interested in health and fitness at all. However, at a commercial gym, the members are people who are already paying a fee to have a membership at the gym and are therefore obviously interested in their health and fitness,

The protocol discussed in this book will be less effective in smaller or boutique gyms with small numbers of gym members simply due to having a smaller pool of potential clients.

INTRODUCTION

MOTH TO FLAME

AN OFFLINE LEAD GENERATION PROTOCOL FOR NEW PERSONAL TRAINERS

INTRODUCTION

ABOUT ME

My relationship with the gym started in my first year at university where I was studying sport and exercise psychology and I also joined the American football team as a running back in that first year.

American football is a fun sport, but it's even more fun if you can hit as hard as you get hit. I was a very skinny 18-year-old at the time, so I knew I had to put on some size. I started going to the gym with a friend I made on the first day of class, who became my teammate and gym partner.

I later stopped playing American football at the end of my second year at university but my habit of going to the gym stuck and I continued to train throughout my time at university.

Fast forward to graduating from university, I started working at the head office of one of the UK's most popular commercial gyms where a lot of personal trainers also worked. These personal trainers that worked at the head office with me would often see me at one of the branches of the gym that was directly below the head office. At this point in my fitness journey, I had gotten in pretty good shape and knew how to train, so naturally they would often encourage me to become a personal trainer any time the subject came up.

After a year of hearing "you should become a Personal trainer", I took the plunge and booked onto a course. In 2016 I became qualified, started working immediately and the rest is history.

I worked at that first gym for 3 years after which I did some further training which led to me stopping my personal training business and working as a diabetes practitioner for the national health service where I helped diabetic patients with their diet and exercise. I then later restarted my business at a different gym but this time I was working as a diabetes practitioner by day and a personal trainer by night.

At different points in this book, I reference the fact that I was not a massive user of social media, in that

I never took the time to build a following on social media platforms, this is partly due to my upbringing.

I was born in Nigeria and moved over to England in my early teens, the internet and phone were not a thing in my world growing up. However, this is only partly a reason, I'm sure there are plenty of people in the same situation as me who flourished on social media. I just never took to it and wasn't particularly interested in posting every day to build a following.

I did create an Instagram account for my personal training, on which I posted sporadically, something for potential clients who are curious about my services to look at, a form of online CV.

Ultimately, I knew if I wasn't going to make the effort on social media, then I had to make the effort somewhere else, I needed a way to generate leads and develop a client base and I tried a few different things before developing the "Moth to Flame" protocol.

PRE MOTH TO FLAME

MOTH TO FLAME

AN OFFLINE LEAD GENERATION PROTOCOL FOR NEW PERSONAL TRAINERS

PRE MOTH TO FLAME

In the world of online sales, advertisers often put people through what is known as a sales funnel. It is a journey that potential customers go through from prospecting to sales to upselling.

Sales funnels often have what is known as a "Low-ticket offer" item, these items are designed to make it easier for people to say yes and get those prospects into your funnel. They provide an easy way to get people into your sales funnel where they can familiarise themselves with you and build trust in you and your service. It is from that point that you can then introduce them to other products or services you may be providing. It becomes much easier for people in your funnel to say yes to your other services because they are already familiar with you and built up some trust in comparison to your competitors.

The "The Moth to Flame" protocol was somewhat of a "low-ticket offer" item for my personal training business.

My First 3 Years as A Personal Trainer

Before delving into the "Moth to Flame" protocol for personal training business sales, allow me to first give a back story of how it came about and how it evolved over the years into being a sales approach.

In my last year of university, a friend and I went to a kickboxing class just to try it out. We had said at the beginning of the year that we'd try a bunch of new things and kickboxing turned out to be one of them. It was a lot of fun and a great workout, but we never went back.

At the time I was two years into lifting, and I was more focused on making "gains" than cardio. I'm unsure of what my friend's initial motivations were at the time but neither of us went back to that particular kickboxing gym, but it had left an impression on me.

Years later, when I became a personal trainer, I read the book "Ignite the Fire", like most information you will find online regarding building up your personal training business, it spoke about having a niche, something that sets you slightly apart from other personal trainers in your gym or local area.

So, I looked at my gym, looked at what other personal trainers were doing, and I decided that as well as personal training, I would add kickboxing cardio sessions as a part of my offering and another string to my bow to differentiate from other PTs as nobody else was doing kickboxing at my gym at the time.

Remember I mentioned that my friend and I never returned to the kickboxing gym after that one class? Well, I knew that I had to know enough about kickboxing if I wanted to offer this to clients, so I went to a few more kickboxing classes to get more familiar with the various kickboxing moves, teaching points, and familiarise myself with pad holding effectively to make sure I can deliver the sessions safely. I had no intention of turning anyone into kickboxing champions but even as a tool for cardio purposes, it was still important to learn more and know enough to confidently run the sessions.

Deciding to offer kickboxing H.I.I.T cardio to anyone interested was a starting point, but unfortunately it by no means meant that suddenly all the gym members were knocking at my door or forming lines because I had decided on a niche. I wish it was that easy but no, I still had to figure out exactly what I was going to do to get new clients and fill my diary.

I tried a number of different things to generate leads and pick up new clients with varying degrees of success. When I look back, I would now describe my initial approaches to gaining new clients as passive, although I did not think so at the time. It wasn't until one specific event happened, this event was the catalyst that changed my approach and attitude towards personal training business sales and gaining new clients, it was something I wasn't doing and something nobody else at my gym was doing at the time. I will be talking about what this catalyst was in later parts of the book.

As I mentioned earlier, I tried a number of different approaches to generating leads and picking up new clients with varying degrees of success, but there was some success.

Scan the QR Code Below to view some of the clients I was working with during that period of time. This will take you to an Instagram page where you can view a promotional video I made with my clients at the time.

I had a good base of clients at any specific time, however looking back, I still didn't feel in control of my business and I would still consider my methods of picking up these clients as slow and passive compared to the "Moth to Flame" Protocol.

Other Ways I Picked Up Clients

I will now discuss some of the other methods I tried to help generate leads and pick up clients in my first 3 years as a personal trainer.

1. Offering taster sessions after group classes.

The setup of some gyms may be different but for most commercial gyms in the UK (and I would assume a similar format in other parts of the world is pretty common), you have the option to join the gym as an "**Hours**" **PT** or as a "**Rent**" **PT.**

Being on hours means that you typically work 15 hours per week for the gym, teaching classes, helping members, and getting annoyed at people for not putting their weights back. Outside your 15 hours of work for the gym, you then get to train your clients and typically keep all the profits for yourself.

If you join as a Rent PT, that means you go straight to paying a fixed monthly rent payment to run your personal training business from the gym and use the equipment. As of the time of writing this, rent payment is typically around £500 to £1,000 per month in the UK depending on location.

When starting out as a personal trainer with no client base, I would 100% recommend starting on hours. You get to familiarise yourself with gym members and build relationships. This is by no means the only way to get started, I know personal trainers who have gone straight into a boutique gym, but in my experience, those are people that already have a wide network of people either in their general life or via social media.

Should you stay on hours? That's completely up to you and your life circumstances.

If you have a kid and family, you may decide that you want your 15 hours back, or as your business grows you may decide you would rather pay the monthly rent and personal train in those hours instead, you'd make the money back and much more.

However, if you don't want to be on rent, it's important to make the most of the 15 hours on the gym floor to promote yourself and your business.

Where most personal trainers go wrong is they spend their 15 hours standing around and putting weights back. Don't get me wrong, put the weights back and tidy the gym, but do it as quickly as possible so that you have more time to speak to gym members and build your business, every single interaction counts, and someone you casually spoke to on the gym floor today could become your client in 3 months. When you speak to gym members, even just for casual conversation, you become a familiar face and they are more likely to come to you with other questions, the more comfortable they get with you the higher the potential of them becoming a future client.

The most beneficial part of being a hours personal trainer, is getting in front of gym members to teach classes, all participants in your class are potential clients and you should deliver your classes as such.

I saw class participants as members who already see the value of following a plan that someone else has created for them, they probably value the motivation that comes from being in a class and may feel that they would not stick to their workout or even come to the gym if not for the classes. I came to realise that as far as target audiences go, I don't believe a better one exists in a gym environment.

After starting as a personal trainer in a commercial gym, one of the first things I noticed other personal trainers did was sometimes offer a "free taster" session to class participants after the class.

It would go something like this:

"I have had 3 personal training slots open up and I am currently offering free personal training taster sessions/consultations to individuals looking to transform their lose weight. If you have any questions regarding your fitness goals or if you are interested in personal training, please stay behind after the class for a quick chat".

I then noticed that PTs would have either their business cards or a board for people to write down their names and contact details or speak to people directly after the class.

So, I did the same and I certainly picked up some clients from doing so in the first few years.

Pro Tip:

The best time to make this announcement is after the workout has ended but before the cool-down stretch.

Typically, when a workout finishes, you may give people a minute or so to catch their breath before going into a cool-down stretch.

I found this little gap to be the best time to make such an announcement. If you try to make this announcement after the class, you will find that as soon as the stretching is done or even before, people are already leaving the class and you then have to announce the fact that you want to make an announcement just to get people to stay and listen, and some people will be gone before you get the chance.

If you make the announcement before the stretch, people are waiting patiently for the cool-down stretch to begin and you still have their full attention. In that gap, you can make your announcement and go straight into the cool-down stretch, nice and smooth.

If you make the announcement at the beginning of the class and then put people through an intense workout, the chances are that they would have completely forgotten about your taster session by the end of the workout.

I also found giving people your business card to be a waste of time for the simple fact that people do not take action. We all procrastinate, I do it, you do it and they most definitely will do it too when it comes to reaching out to you, you want to keep control of the process as much as possible.

I found some success by getting people to write their names and contact details and then reaching out to those people to have a conversation and book a consultation or taster session.

There is already familiarity and some level of trust built between you and your class attendees, I believe this approach was more successful than others for this reason.

2. I tried gym challenges.

Over time, I realized that it was important to have a consistent method of generating new leads.

One of the ways I tried to do this was by conducting gym challenges on a monthly basis with members on the gym floor.

I tried to keep these as fun as possible and actually make them a challenge to incite some competition and draw more people in. One example you can see in the picture below.

In this particular case, the challenge was to connect the dots on the board without the pen leaving the board or going over the same lines twice.

The prize was either a 30-minute weight training taster session or a 30-minute kickboxing taster.

I remember people being very curious about what the challenge was, and it even drew in a crowd of people who wanted to see if the person currently attempting to do the challenge would successfully connect the dots, and some of those later had a go at it themselves.

This was a great way to speak and connect with gym members and speak to more gym members and get them to be more familiar with me as a PT and I did generate a few leads from doing this.

Try it yourself.

Rule: Using only 4 straight lines, connect all 9 dots.

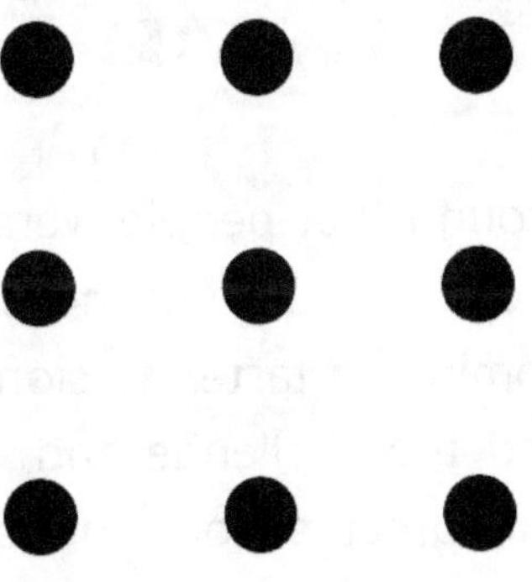

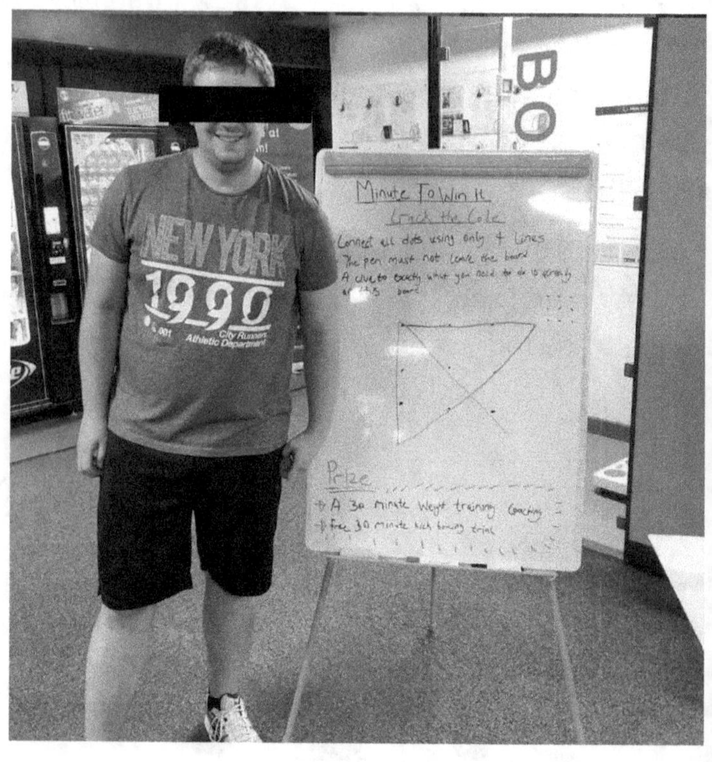

In the end, I found that people were drawn to the challenge more for the sake of the challenge. And I had people coming to taster sessions just because they completed the challenge and won the prize. Even people in great shape who didn't (in their minds at least) feel like they needed a personal trainer took part, some of whom won the challenge.

It meant that I ran a few taster sessions to the wrong audience.

It wasn't a targeted approach.

3. I created gym surveys.

I created gym surveys as a way to generate leads, I approached gym members on their way in or out of the gym and asked them to take a minute of their time to fill out the survey (you should of course not approach people to do this in the middle of their work out).

The design of the gym survey questions (which I created myself) then leads the conversation toward things that the gym offered and promoted to members, such as inductions, free gym classes, free first-time use of massage chairs, free first-time use of the gym's body composition machine and personal training services. These were all the services that the gym offered, and I included them in the survey. As you may be able to guess, I was interested only in the personal training aspect of the survey.

If a member did mention that they were interested in using the services of a personal trainer, they were then able to leave their contact details.

(See an example survey on the next page)

PRODUCT AND SERVICES SURVEY

1. Name (*optional*): ██████████████████████

2. Member Since: _2015_

3. Member at any other gym?   Yes ☐   No ☑

4. If yes, please specify: _______________

5. Did you take an induction after joining?   Yes ☑   No ☐

6. Do you take advantage of the free classes: Yes ☑   No, not yet ☐

7. Have you taken advantage of your **first time free use** of the massage chairs?

   Yes ☐   No, not yet ☑

8. Have you taken advantage of your **first time free use** of the Boditrax precision body composition machine?

   Yes ☐   No, not yet ☑

9. Have you ever considered the help of one of our personal trainers?

   Yes, I could use some pointers ☐   No, I am on track with my goals ☑

10. If yes, would you like to be contacted for a free consultation?

   Yes, I'd like to take action ☑   No ☐

11. If yes, please provide contact details below:

   Email: ████████████████████

   Tel: ████████████████

The picture above shows an example of the survey that a member filled out.

I generated A LOT of leads using the above survey, it is low effort on the member's part and takes roughly about 1 minute for gym members to complete.

So, when I approached members of the gym on their way in and out and said:

"Hello, do you mind filling out this gym survey, it'll take you less than a minute".

Most people were happy to take a minute to fill it out.

<u>Pro Tip:</u>

Despite generating a high number of leads, I only remember converting two members into actual clients.

In hindsight, I believe this was down to my approach to contacting the members. I typically emailed or texted people, which left things in the hands of the member to get back to me and a lot did not.

If I was to use this approach again, I would call the member directly to discuss why they feel they currently need the services of a personal trainer and try to book them in for a consultation right there on the phone call.

4. I left out consultation boards on the gym floor.

I left out a sign-up board on the gym floor with my availability for people to write their initials in a time slot they wanted and also contact me to confirm.

GRINDDNA KICK FIT – A kickboxing fitness program

CLAIM YOUR 30 MINUTE TASTER SESSION NOW!

	7 – 7:30 am	7:30 – 8 am	8:30 – 9 am	9 – 9:30 am	10am – 3pm	4 – 4:30 pm	4:30 – 5 pm	5 – 5:30 pm	5:30 – 6 pm	6 – 6:30 pm	6:30 – 7 pm	7 – 7:30 pm
Monday 12th of December												
Tuesday 13th of December												
Wednesday 14th of December												
Thursday 15th of December												
Friday 16th of December												
Saturday 17th of December												

Instructions:

1. Write your name/initials in an available slot above
2. [illegible] with your name and the time you would like

Want more information or have other personal Training Enquiries? Get in touch on:

/administrating   /grinddna

At the bottom of the board, it said:

Instructions:

1. Write your name/initials in an available time slot above.

2. Text *contact number* with your name and the time you have chosen.

This is an approach I took right at the beginning of my personal training career, literally a few months in.

I do not remember getting any clients or even leads from doing this.

Pro Tip:

Do not do this, at least not in this way, it was a waste of time.

Looking back, the reason this approach wasn't successful is obvious. First, I am asking them to stop and write their name on the board, and then pull out their phone and text me a date and time.

It left too much in the hands of the member to do and as I mentioned before, people do not take action.

You may start to notice a running theme.

5. I created a pull-up banner and quiz.

Another lead generation approach I took was creating a huge banner that stood near the entrance of the gym in clear view of people to see on their way in and out of the gym.

(See the banner on the next page)

I then had a quiz form that people filled in and submitted into a box for me to later review.

I had a picture of one of my client transformations on the banner to grab people's attention and interest with the aim of getting people to participate in the quiz and generate leads.

The quiz people were required to complete was designed to expose their knowledge gaps, to which I offered them a consultation to help fill these knowledge gaps. Point 3, also states that they will be provided with a customised gym routine to help achieve their weight loss goals.

This meant that for people who took the quiz and were interested in what was on offer, they would then need to provide their details for me to get in touch.

This approach led to a few consultations over time, two of which turned into paying clients.

Looking back, I would again say this was passive and left too much in the hands of the members. In these examples, the client has to decide to take part in the quiz, decide to leave their details and when you contact them, they have to decide if the quiz they completed in the spur of the moment was still something that they cared enough about.

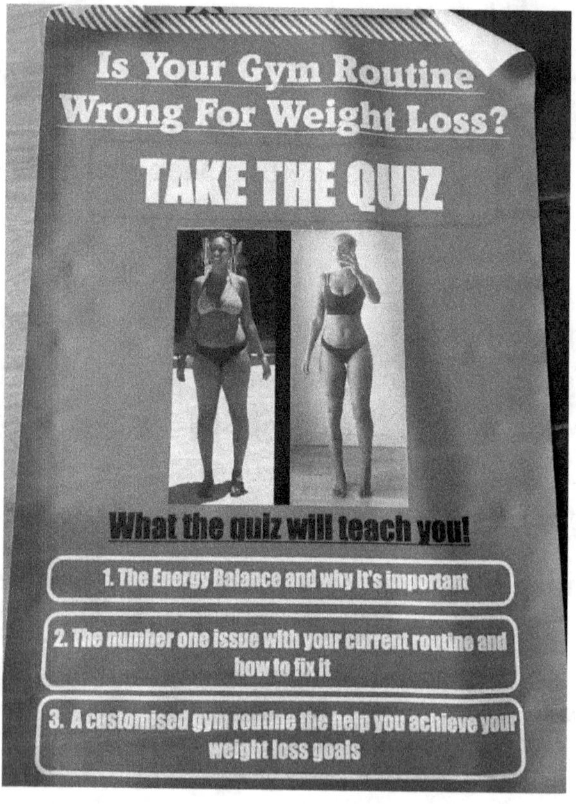

As with some of the other methods I tried, most people did not get back in touch after contacting them.

As I pointed out in a previous example, the best contact method is to call the member directly to have a conversation over the phone.

This is a lesson I had not learned at the time, and it affected how successful my efforts were.

6. I distributed goody bags to corporate offices around my gym with a call-to-action flyer.

My gym at the time was located in the city centre of my city (or "Downtown" if you're an American reading this"). This meant there were a lot of corporate offices all around my gym.

One week, I went around the corporate offices early in the morning and distributed a goody bag to people as they were entering the building.

In the goody bag was a flyer with some useful tips for office workers on one side and on the other side, there were pictures of body transformations from two of my clients at the time. And a call to action.

What was the outcome of this? NOTHING.

Not a single thing, no leads, therefore no clients.

Is it possible that one of the people that received a goody bag from me later became a client without me realising their first point of contact with me was the goody bag? sure, but I had no one reach out directly as a result of this approach.

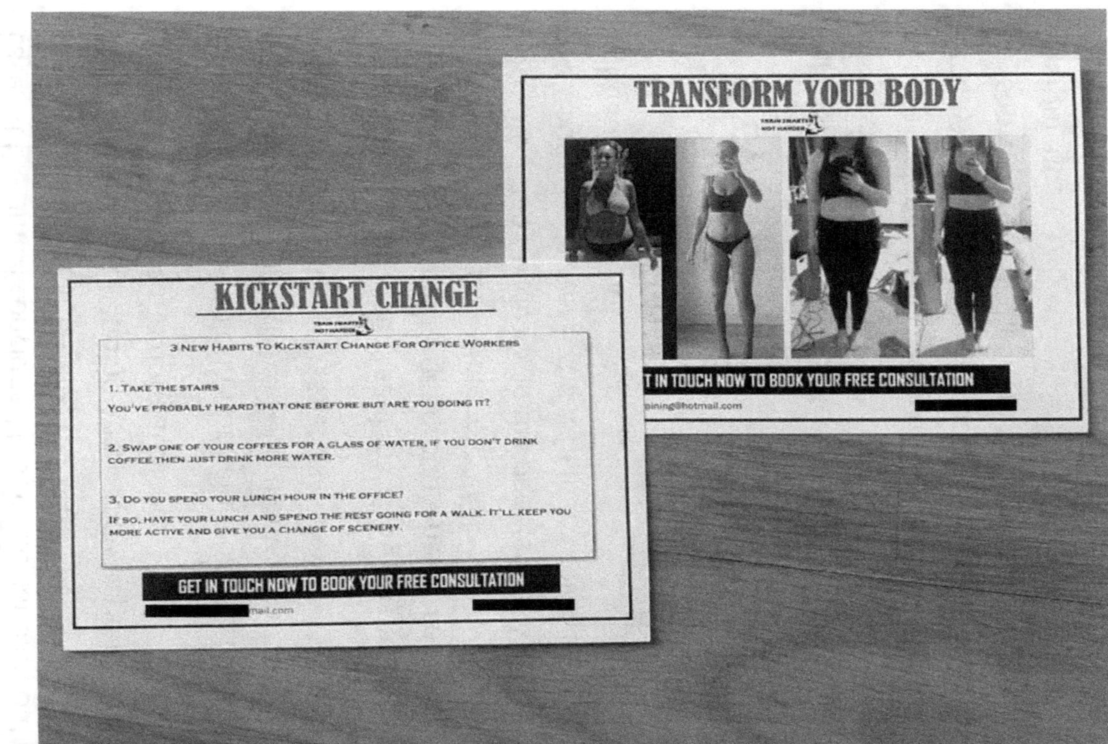
KICKSTART CHANGE
TRAIN SMARTER NOT HARDER
3 New Habits To Kickstart Change For Office Workers
1. Take the stairs
You've probably heard that one before but are you doing it?
2. Swap one of your coffees for a glass of water, if you don't drink coffee then just drink more water.
3. Do you spend your lunch hour in the office?
If so, have your lunch and spend the rest going for a walk. It'll keep you more active and give you a change of scenery.
GET IN TOUCH NOW TO BOOK YOUR FREE CONSULTATION
mail.com
TRANSFORM YOUR BODY
TRAIN SMARTER NOT HARDER
GET IN TOUCH NOW TO BOOK YOUR FREE CONSULTATION
mining@hotmail.com

I remember analysing why that might have been the case. At the time, I concluded that while handing out the goody bags at the corporate offices, I had no idea whom I was handing the goody bags to and whether they were the right audience.

There were just people in normal or office clothing who may or may not have been members of a gym or even interested in fitness at all.

Remember earlier when I said that the gym members in a class are a good target group when it comes to targeting the right audience, well this was the opposite. I had no idea who the people that received the goody bags were and whether they were the right audience or not.

7. Gym inductions

This one is pretty simple and straightforward, commercial gyms typically have inductions for people looking to join the gym and people who have already joined the gym can book a gym induction to be shown around the gym and how to use the equipment.

When I began working as a personal trainer, I would volunteer to do as many inductions as possible, whether I was the personal trainer on shift at the time or not.

Why are gym inductions a great opportunity for picking up clients?

If you think about the kind of person that signs up for an induction, it's likely to be someone who has just joined a gym or is looking to join a gym but doesn't know what they are doing or doesn't feel confident around the gym.

Rarely would you have an experienced gym goer who would sign up for a gym induction. If you're experienced with the gym, it can be safe to assume that you know how to use the basic gym equipment and it's likely that you simply join, turn up and just walk around to see how the equipment is laid out.

I found the people that signed up for gym inductions are typically people who weren't familiar with the gym and the equipment and wanted to be shown their way around both.

Showing people around the gym is a great opportunity to have a conversation to find out why they have decided to join, what their goals are, how experienced they are with the gym, and whether or not they feel they need any help moving towards their goals, and that's where you and your personal training services come in.

Pro Tip:

Treat gym inductions as consultations/taster sessions that didn't require any lead generation on your part.

You would be surprised how many "hours" personal trainers look at the tasks they are required to do whilst doing their 15 hours as just that, tasks they have to do.

Instead, you should look at gym inductions, classes, and the parading of the gym floor all as opportunities to build your business.

These are a few of the lead generation methods I have tried during my first 3 years at the gym, that is until a catalyst event happened that changed my approach moving forward.

A lot of the methods discussed did generate leads and if I was to attempt them again, the main change I would make would be to call clients directly for a phone conversation instead of texting or emailing.

THE CATALYST

MOTH TO FLAME

AN OFFLINE LEAD GENERATION PROTOCOL FOR NEW PERSONAL TRAINERS

THE CATALYST

In the 3 years I spent at my first gym, I saw many personal trainers come and go. They say 80% of personal trainers fail within the first year, I don't know if that percentage is accurate, but I certainly saw many come and go.

Towards the end of my last year at the first gym, a new personal trainer joined the gym, I've named him the catalyst.

This personal trainer came in and unlike all the others that had been in that gym before, he built his business up so fast and blew past other personal trainers in the gym in very little time.

He didn't promote anything on social media, but he did do one thing that no personal trainer in the gym was doing at the time, including me. That is, to go up directly to gym members to promote his business. Yes, I would see him randomly walk up to someone on the treadmill, have a conversation, and a few days later I would see him having a consultation with that same person who later became his client. He would approach people regularly and consistently and in no time, he had built a better business than most personal trainers at the gym.

The only thing I had on this guy was time, I had built up more business than him because I had been at the gym longer and had a larger client base for that reason.

I was very aware that it took me much longer to build up my business and client base (using my passive approaches discussed earlier) to the same level that he managed to build his up to in just a few months.

Prior to this personal trainer coming into the gym, I would say that I was one of the more active personal trainers at my gym in terms of making lead generation a part of my business, it's easy to just focus on training your clients, it's the reason you became a personal trainer and many fell into the trap of just training their clients and then out of nowhere, three clients have drop off and they have a dent in their earnings and no leads

Despite actively making lead generation a part of my business I had to reassess my approach because what I did in a year, I saw someone else do in less than 6 months.

Whilst I had a board out somewhere on the gym floor waiting for people to fill in a quiz, contacting those leads and getting no response from most. I saw someone else speaking to multiple people directly on the gym floor, having consultations a few days later with multiple of those people, and building his client base. Suddenly my efforts felt passive.

This was a new personal trainer, not just to my gym but to personal training as a whole, that was clear to see in other aspects of his coaching, but he was keen to learn and would ask questions about other aspects of personal training that he wasn't sure about but I could see very clearly that his approach to promoting his business was something he had a good handle on.

It's important to note that my observations of him generated feelings of inspiration and not envy, I was watching someone with much less experience do something in a much better way, and I felt that if he can do it, so could I. I was inspired to take a new approach with my lead generation.

When such an individual walks into the gym, you can either lean away and decide they have nothing to teach you because you are a more experienced personal trainer, or you lean in and see what you can learn from what you can see happening in front of you.

There is a question that my parents would always ask me as a child in such a situation, that question is "do they have two heads?" Meaning, whatever you see other people do, whatever success people are having, you are capable of it too because they don't have two heads, they have one head and one brain just like you, so figure it out.

Being someone that is huge on personal development, I'm always open to an opportunity to improve in any way, so, I leaned in and allowed myself to be inspired by his actions and approach.

The truth is most personal trainers would rather do a hundred things before approaching people randomly on the gym floor, not just to chit chat but to directly promote their business. They say, "The cave you fear to enter holds the treasure you seek", well approaching and directly promoting your business to clients on the gym floor is a cave that most personal trainers refuse to enter.

They also say, "Seeing is believing". After seeing how much faster he was able to build up his business in comparison to my approach, I was sold on making an effort to be more direct.

This is the beginning of my development the approach I now refer to as "Moth to Flame" protocol.

SIDE NOTE

Whilst writing this, the phrase "Comparison is the thief of joy" came to mind. It's important for me to note to readers that there is a difference between comparing yourself to someone and comparing an approach/a business tactic or looking at what another business is doing and seeing how it can benefit your business.

My comparison was not between myself and the catalyst as people but rather between his approach to lead generation vs mine.

This is an important distinction.

MOTH TO

FLAME

MOTH TO FLAME

AN OFFLINE LEAD GENERATION PROTOCOL FOR NEW PERSONAL TRAINERS

MOTH TO FLAME

After deciding that I needed to ditch my boards and quizzes and start approaching members on the gym floor to promote my business and make an offer. I decided that I needed something specific to approach members with.

I didn't want to go up to members on the gym floor to correct their form and try to sell them personal training from there, that wasn't an appealing approach to me.

I needed a specific and structured approach that I can repeat pretty much all the time, I needed a system.

Whilst I was an "hours" personal trainer, one of my most popular classes was called combat, which is essentially just shadow kickboxing. It was also by far one of the most popular classes at the gym and probably at most gyms.

I also knew that my clients at the time loved it when we did kickboxing for cardio as part of our training session, so I knew that it's something that people love to do and take part in.

However, I had never promoted kickboxing in a direct way to gym members. So, I decided I would create a kickboxing-only H.I.I.T program to offer clients and directly approach people on the gym floor with some sort of structure to my approach. I knew kickboxing was something fun that people liked to do for cardio but at the time, I wasn't sure how well my new plan would actually work.

In the sections below I will talk about the first iteration of the "Moth to Flame" approach, some of the tweaks I made, and how this first iteration (Version 1) transitioned to Version 2 and became a "low-ticket" funnel item that later led to personal training clients and helped me go from £0 to £2,000 in 9 weeks when I moved to a different gym with zero clients.

Moth to Flame V1

The Plan

As I mentioned, I decided to offer a service that was just kickboxing.

The offer was simple, 2 x 30-minute H.I.I.T kickboxing cardio sessions per week.

Both 30-minute sessions had to be completed in the same week, so clients could <u>not</u> do one 30-minute session this week and another the following week.

I set things out in this way because it meant that each kickboxing client would at least equate to the same as having one regular personal training client on a one-session-per-week package.

Clients would be required to pay for the full hour, meaning no payments were accepted for a 30-minute session and payment for sessions was collected on a monthly basis using a direct debit system called "GoCardless", the importance of having payment collection set up in an automatic manner could be a subject all on its own.

After showing clients an effective warm-up and cool-down routine, clients would be required to do the warm-up before the session and cool down after the session by themselves, this is so that we can make the most of the 30-minute session. An intense 30-minute kickboxing H.I.I.T session is an amazing workout, and I knew that because I already did kickboxing for cardio with some of my weight training clients.

Splitting the 1 hour into two sessions also made the clients feel like they were getting more for their money, and they were, it was an easy sell.

For myself, I would make sure to always schedule the sessions around other PT sessions so that I was never coming into the gym just for a 30-minute session.

The Execution

To execute, I started to approach members of the gym with a very specific goal in mind.

I had a script, and I followed it.

So, I am going to create a roleplay scenario below of a typical approach:

I am standing on the gym floor looking around.

Since the kickboxing session was aimed at cardio, I would aim my script in that direction and tweak it slightly to match the situation.

<u>Example Scenario 1</u>

A member is on a cardio machine but not in an intense workout.

For example, a member casually cycling on the exercise bike, a member walking on the treadmill or casually using any cardio equipment.

In this scenario, I would walk up next to the exercise bike, or stand on the neighbouring treadmill and the conversation would go something like this:

<u>Me</u>: "Hello, I have a question for you."

(Saying this in the first sentence makes the gym member curious about what question you could possibly have for them, and it grabs their attention)

<u>Gym member:</u> "Hello, yeah, what's up?"

<u>Me</u>: "I can see you're obviously doing some cardio at the moment, is cardio a regular part of your gym routine?"

They might say something along the lines:

<u>Gym Member:</u> "Yeah, I try and do a bit here and there.

Then I say:

<u>Me</u>: "Okay, that's good! I'm running some kickboxing H.I.I.T <u>trial</u> sessions at the moment <u>for</u> <u>cardio purposes</u>, have you ever done any kickboxing before?

(Pay attention to the <u>underlined</u> words above as I will be discussing the significance of having these words as part of the script)

They might say:

<u>Gym member:</u> "No, I've never done any kickboxing actually, but it looks fun."

Or

"Yeah, I tried it once a long time ago, I really enjoyed it."

Whatever the response is, I then say:

<u>**Me:**</u> "It's a great way to have a full body H.I.I.T. workout and tone up whilst learning some self-defence moves as well, and it's a lot more fun than the treadmill (or whatever cardio machine they're on at the time). Is it something you would like to try?"

The response I received the most to this offer was a yes. Most people said yes, and they said yes with enthusiasm.

What I did next, after the gym member has said yes turned out to be VERY important and affected my conversation from that person saying yes to them actually turning up for the trial.

I only realised how important it was through trial and error and I will speak about this further down in this section.

But before I do, remember the underlined words above that I said were important to keep in the script? Let's talk about them briefly.

First is making sure to call the session a **trial** and here's why:

Originally, my script would say that I am running some free kickboxing taster sessions, naturally, this came from offering free taster sessions for personal training, so I naturally applied the same language.

However, I noticed a huge difference when I labelled it as a trial.

Psychologically, we have all had trials of a product or service and we are psychologically primed to expect that a free trial typically comes with the expectation that you continue with the product or service if you are happy with it.

I could see a difference when I started to refer to the sessions as a trial both at the initial approach and after the session.

During the initial approach, the difference I could see is in the follow-up questions that people would have.

People would ask me:

"How does it work after the trial?"

"How much do the normal sessions cost?"

These were not questions that I received when I referred to the sessions as a "free taster session". These follow-up questions showed that I was setting up the right intentions and expectations for the people that did come along to the trial sessions. This definitely led to a better conversion of the gym member into a kickboxing H.I.I.T. client after the trial.

This is important and should not be ignored as it will affect your results.

Secondly, I would make sure that my script included the phrase "**for cardio purposes**".

I wanted to be clear on the purpose of the sessions, i.e., a fun way to do cardio and improve on cardiovascular fitness.

My reasoning behind stating that is simple, I am not a kickboxing world champion, and neither was I trying to turn them into one.

My interest in martial arts grew more and more naturally over the years. Fast forward to today, where I train Muay Thai weekly and have had a few fights, but at the time I knew a handful of kickboxing techniques and enough creativity to have a safe and fun workout.

This is again about setting expectations and making sure the gym member is clear on what you are offering.

<u>Example Scenario 2</u>

A member is on the gym floor.

Maybe on their way in or out.

I approached members anywhere I came across them in the gym, with the exception of anyone intensely working out, whether that's cardio or weights.

Why? Well, if they're between sets of intense lifts, they're probably out of breath and can't/don't want to speak to you.

If they are intensely working out on a cardio machine, well that should be self-explanatory. You would be wasting your time trying to talk to someone running on a treadmill or going crazy on a bike or even someone trying to catch their breath in-between sets.

If you look at a simple scenario, someone walking into the gym, or someone walking from the changing rooms towards the gym floor.

The only difference in my approach would be a slight change in the phrasing of my words.

Before I even say anything, the first part of my approach would be to gain the individual's attention.

If the person is on the gym floor, it's likely they are on the move unlike if they are on a cardio machine.

So, to stop them in their tracks, a simple wave to gain their attention worked just fine, once I get their attention enough for them to make eye contact, I would immediately say:

<u>Me</u>: "Hello, I have a question for you"

<u>Gym member:</u> "Hello, yeah, what's up?"

<u>Me:</u> "Do you do a lot of cardio as part of your training?"

In this scenario, I have no idea what this person does at the gym, so I first try to determine if the member is a good fit by simply asking the question.

The two likely responses to the question are something along the lines of:

<u>Gym Member:</u> "Yes, I usually do some sprints, or I go running sometimes"

Or

<u>Gym Member:</u> "No, I usually don't, I mainly focus on weight training"

If the gym member says yes, I simply follow the same steps as scenario 1.

If the gym member says no, it's likely that they would follow up with "Why do you ask?" and even if they don't say it out loud, they are most likely curious about your reason for asking that question.

So even if the gym member says no, my response would be along the lines of:

Me: "Ah okay, I see. The reason I ask is that I am running some kickboxing H.I.I.T trial sessions at the moment for cardio purposes but if you don't do much cardio then it may not be a good fit for you at this time".

To which the member might say:

- "Yeah, not at the moment"

However, I have had multiple situations where the member responded with an enthusiastic

- "Oh really? I've always wanted to try kickboxing."

In which case I would ask if they wanted to try it and that could lead to another yes.

In either scenario, if the gym member says no, I simply respond with "No worries at all, have a nice workout".

What To Do After The "Yes".

Now let's talk about what I did after the gym member said, "Yes, I would like to have a trial of the session".

Well initially, I took down their name and phone number and sent them a text. In doing this, I very quickly ran into the same problems as I did in other lead-generation methods I had tried before. A lot of people would not get back in touch after reaching out, or they have to check this other plan they have first before they can confirm a date, or something came up and they're not sure when they can do the session, or some other type of barrier would pop up.

On my end, I found that communicating with 15 to 20 people in an attempt to get them booked in for a session the following week proved difficult and messy.

What I did to get around this was to take down the gym member's name and number and also book them into an agreed time slot right there and then.

So, I downloaded a calendar app on my phone and when the gym member said yes to the trial session, I would pull out my phone, show them the calendar and my current available slots and ask them which time slot that week or the following week works best for them.

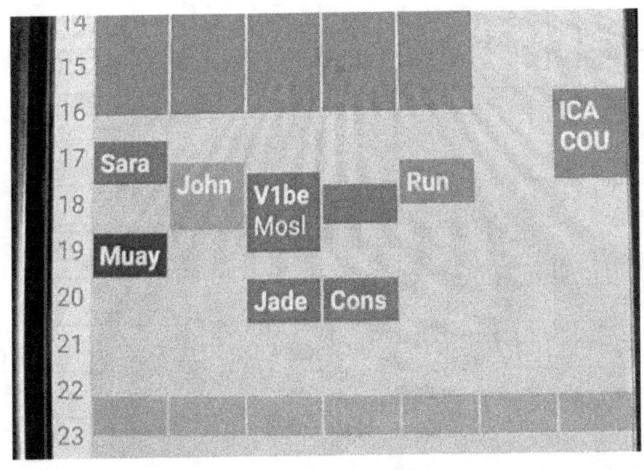

They would pick a time slot and watch me add them to my diary and I would say, "Perfect, I'll see you then".

I would then later send them a text simply confirming the session and the date and time agreed.

It would read:

*"Hello *insert name*.*

It was nice to meet you earlier today.

*I have booked you in for your H.I.I.T kickboxing trial session next Tuesday the *insert date* at 2:30 pm.*

If you have any questions, please let me know.

See you then 😊 "

The day before the session, I would send another text as a reminder,

It would read:

*"Hello *<u>insert name</u>".*

This is a reminder for your kickboxing trial session tomorrow at 2:30 pm.

If you have any questions, please let me know.

Looking forward to seeing you then."

This slight change in my approach worked like a charm to make a huge difference and psychology can tell us why.

Have you ever wondered why you have to opt out of Organ donation (at least in the UK)? Meaning you are automatically considered to agree to donate your organs when you die unless you record a decision to opt-out. You may have also noticed that on some websites you have to opt out of receiving marketing emails, otherwise, you are automatically assumed to agree.

Kurt Lewin, a German American psychologist who is often referred to as the father of American social psychology was a key contributor in the field of social psychology. One of his key contributions was a simple change of strategy to create behaviour change amongst people, this was called "The Lewinian Recipe".

The Lewinian Recipe in the "Moth to Flames" Approach.

Lewin stated:

"Make the actions you want to encourage easier, akin to moving downhill: and make the actions you want to discourage more difficult, akin to moving uphill."

In the book "The Wisest One in the Room" Authors Thomas Gilovich and Lee Ross talked about a great example of Lewin's recipe manifesting itself. In the book, they talked about a study that examined organ donation rates in European countries with different default donation policies.

Countries with an opt-in policy required individuals to take some action, such as signing the back of their driver's license. Without this signature, the person's organs cannot be used for someone in need.

In other countries, the default is reversed. All individuals are considered potential donors unless they sign the back of their license to indicate otherwise, they had to take action to opt-out.

The study found that countries with an opt-out policy had participation rates of nearly 100%, while participation rates in countries with an opt-in policy were on average about 15%.

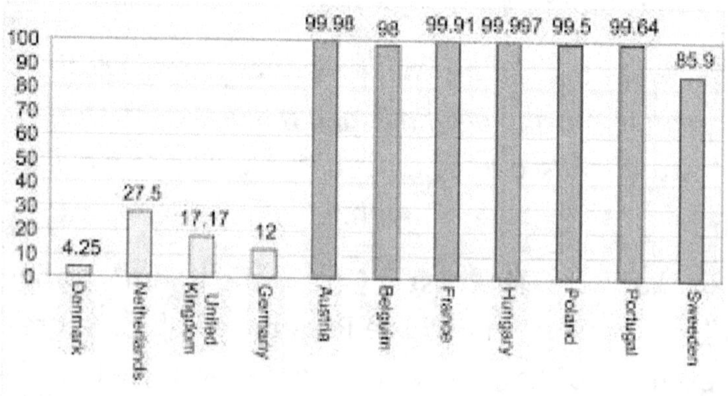

Difference in organ donation rates in EU countries with an opt-in policy (Green) and an opt-out policy (Purple)

Making the government's desired behaviour (having more organ donors) the default behaviour meant that countries with an opt-out policy had no barriers in the way of being an organ donor.

The same effect was at play during my process of booking people in for their trial session. With my original approach, whereby I was contacting people to arrange a time and date, I was essentially asking people to opt-in and the success rate was low.

In contrast, when I started booking people in for their trial on the spot and sending a text simply as confirmation. They at that point became automatically opted in and cancelling the trial then becomes the more difficult action. For that reason, I experienced a much higher turnout to the trial sessions, which of course leads to more conversions to clients.

With this structure and these tweaks, I was well on my way to implementing this new approach to my lead generation.

I had a structured and repeatable game plan and in no time, I too was walking up to complete strangers at the gym, having a consultation with them within a few days to a week of our first conversation, and turning many of those into paying clients. It was the fastest and most successful way I had ever attempted in picking new clients.

It was like I was waving a flame in a fleet of moths.

Most importantly, I felt like I had complete control of my business, and I knew that from that point if I needed to pick up new clients I could go and get it by speaking to enough people, I didn't have to wait for them to come to me.

Moth To Flame V2

After implementing this protocol and running the H.I.I.T. kickboxing cardio sessions with the clients that I had picked up, I started to notice a few things.

Those clients would often ask me about personal training or talk to me about what else they were doing at the gym. They would have a lot of questions, which led to requests for weight training programs from some or requests for weight training sessions in addition to the H.I.I.T kickboxing sessions from others. Of course, I obliged and a lot of the H.I.I.T kickboxing clients that I had either eventually did some weight training alongside the H.I.I.T kickboxing session or they switched completely over to weight training.

I noticed it was very easy to 'upsell' or convert my kickboxing clients into regular personal training clients. At the time, this was all happening organically at the request of the clients with no conscious push from me. This later changed when I moved to a different gym, and I began to treat the process as a lead generation and funnel system.

Before switching to a different gym, I had made some slight career changes. After working at my first commercial gym for three years, I decided to venture into other parts of the health and fitness world where I could still apply my knowledge and experience.

I started working for the national healthcare system as a diabetes practitioner. Just as well because 6 months later the infamous global pandemic hit, and all the gyms were shut. I considered myself lucky during this period because I was still able to work as a diabetes practitioner by working from home giving diabetic patients guidance about their diets over the phone.

Fast forward to over a year of working from home to the re-opening of gyms. I had decided that as much as I enjoyed working as a diabetes practitioner, I missed working with clients in person, in a social environment.

I made the decision to join a different commercial gym in a different part of the city. It was my first time starting afresh again as a personal trainer with zero client base. I was also in a different part of the city which meant I couldn't just tell my old clients to come to my gym.

I've always felt personal training is a great job because it's one you can do anywhere. So, I took the fresh start as a challenge, I told myself "If personal training is a job that I want to be able to do anywhere, then you need to be able to start afresh anywhere".

So that was my challenge to myself, and I felt that I was experienced enough to make it happen.

My circumstances this time were different because I was also working as a diabetes practitioner, so I set my working hours as 5:30 pm to 8:30 pm, 3 hours per day, five days per week. I was looking for 15 hours of personal training.

I wasted zero time; I had done a bunch of things in the past to get clients but on the first day of entering that new gym, I immediately started approaching gym members with my already tried and tested script.

However, unlike at the previous gym where I already had personal training clients and the H.I.I.T kickboxing sessions were an additional "service" of mine. At this new gym, I had zero clients, and I knew that I wanted some regular resistance training clients.

I remembered how easy it was to convert my H.I.I.T. kickboxing clients into regular personal training clients, so with that in mind I simply added one extra step to my previous system.

The Pre-Trial Consultation

The Pre Trial-Consultation was a 15-to-30-minute conversation that I would have with the potential client immediately before the trial session. I treated it like the normal consultation that I would have with a regular personal training client and filled in the consultation form.

The intention was to be more proactive in finding out which of the potential clients that sign up may benefit from resistance training-focused personal training sessions.

Unlike at the previous gym, where I later found out that the client was also interested in weight training. I decided to approach the conversion of clients from kickboxing into weight training more proactively where it is suited to the client.

Having more information about the client's overall goals allowed me to speak to these clients about transitioning into weight training if it was complimentary to their goals.

Consultation Form

Name:

D.O.B:

What? (3 goals you would like to achieve/ describe your ideal body/ physic)

Describe where you are at now? (body/fitness level and otherwise)

When? (any particular time frame in?)

Why? (why are these goals important to you/ how would it make you feel if you achieved this?)

Current Routine? (what are you doing now to achieve these goals?)

What will be required of you to achieve this....? (My recommendations and discuss ENERGY BALLANCE)

(Discuss... diet/nutrition/NEAT/EAT/cardio/weight training? /calories/types of food/habit and lifestyle changes)

On a scale of 1 to 10... how important is it for you to achieve those goals?

____

Why is it important?

How confident are you that you will be able to achieve your goals? (on a scale of 1 to 10)

____

Why did you say that number?

How would you feel if by set time frame you have not achieved your goals? (so if you don't get on the right nutrition a exercise program and habit changes, how would you feel if you are in the same position or worse)

Plan of Action:

Measurements

Height	
Weight	
Body Fat %	
Waist	
Arms	
Thighs	

Contact Details:

Tel:

Email:

Having these consultations before the trial also meant that in a scenario where the potential client came to the trial but wasn't sure if it was the right thing for them, I am able to spot this because I am clearer on their goals.

For example, I may come across a potential client who said yes to the trial because I said it's a great way to improve their overall fitness and tone up. The potential client may have said yes to this because they want to be fit and maybe they hold body fat in their abdominal regions and feel like they have "a bit of a belly" (as some clients would say), so they also want to tone up.

However, in the consultation, the potential client may also say that they want to have stronger legs and bigger arms and chest. With that information, I would adapt my offer to the client's needs and suggest that a 2-session x per week weight training and 1 session x per week H.I.I.T kickboxing session package would be ideal for them.

Assuming the client signs up for this package, that would have fast-forwarded the process of moving or upselling the client from H.I.I.T Kickboxing to weight training.

In my previous approach, without the pre-trial consultation, the client may have mentioned to me in a session, weeks or months later, that they have been trying to build up their legs and arms in their own time, which may have then led to a conversation about adding some weight training sessions to their package, but this would have taken much longer.

The pre-trial consultation allowed me to start many people on a higher package that included weight training, but it also allowed me to know which of my clients that signed up on a H.I.I.T. kickboxing package only, may be interested in weight training later down the line.

A very important takeaway is, at any one time there are multiple members of the gym who would pay for your service if you approached them with one but may never come and ask you for your service, they may never take action on their own.

Taking a pro-active approach with a low-ticket offer that people can easily say yes to will put your miles ahead of other personal trainers who are waiting for members to reach out to them, I know that because I've been on both sides of the coin.

Once they do say yes, they are essentially in your funnel, and it is then up to you to see exactly what they need and how you can help them with it, it's up to you to build up the trust that will make it much easier for them to take you up on any other service you offer. It was easy to convert kickboxing clients into weight training clients because I delivered a fun and effective kickboxing session every time, helped them towards their goals, answered any other fitness questions they had, and gave them useful advice and tips that they found useful.

Naturally, that builds trust and there is only one place that a client who already trains with you and receives useful information and guidance from you will go for other services relating to their fitness goals.

In 9 weeks, I had filled the 15 hours I had available each week with both weight training and H.I.I.T kickboxing clients, all of which came from the "Moth to Flame" protocol detailed above.

Scan the QR code below to see a video collage of some of my clients in action after moving to the second gym.

The information detailed above are the basic steps that I took to take charge of my lead generation and feel more in control of my business, I then truly felt like I could move to any gym with good foot traffic and build up a successful personal training business.

This is a formula for commercial gyms, it works because of the large number of potential clients that already exist at the gym, hence why you don't need social media.

On the topic of social media, please note that if you can use social media to your advantage, then you should. It's a great tool and it's important to have an online presence in this time and age, but you do not have to rely on it.

The "Moth to Flame" protocol puts you completely in the driver's seat. You know that if you take a specific set of actions, you are likely to get a specific set of results, there is only one thing that can stop you from successfully implementing this strategy, and I will discuss exactly what that is in later chapters.

For now, let's look at why the "moth to flame" protocol was the perfect strategy for me and also give you the opportunity to consider what other strategies could be your "Moth to Flame".

What is your moth to flame?

Kickboxing is great "flame" in the "Moth to Flame" offer because people love kickboxing and boxing. It's always a popular class at gyms and in general if you ask someone if they want to do some kickboxing or boxing, there seems to be excitement or eagerness for it, you will find many boutique boxing and kickboxing studios pop up in major cities for this reason.

People come back for more because the benefits are undeniable, there really is no workout like it, it's a great stress reliever and it comes with many more benefits. From all the actual benefits of kickboxing and boxing, I am also of the opinion that a major reason this format of exercise is so popular is that mentally, it can boost people's confidence and as mentioned in a post by the blog site 'asweatlife': "You feel like a badass".

Kickboxing was a great choice for me personally because I had a genuine interest in martial arts that has now led to me being a regular at my muay thai boxing club, where I spar weekly and so far, had a few interclub fights.

However, even in the beginning, my interest in martial arts was enough for me to go to kickboxing classes to learn more about the sport, the techniques, how to hold pads and pick up on how the coaches at the club ran the classes. This helped immensely when it came to running the sessions with clients.

Past the initial excitement of trialling the session, I also believe that the structure I had set out for the sessions made it easy for people to say yes to signing up for the paid sessions.

Offering to break the 1-hour sessions into two 30-minute-high intensity sessions meant that the clients could get more for their money.

They get to have a kickboxing workout twice a week, have someone to hold them accountable for turning up to the gym twice a week, and also have access to a coach that can answer their questions about other aspects of their fitness goals, twice a week.

This setup had no negative impact on me financially or time-wise, clients are required to pay for a full hour with the understanding that the hour will be broken up into two 30-minute sessions, and payments are then collected monthly. Time-wise, I simply arranged kickboxing sessions back-to-back from one client to the next to make up the hour.

So, the clients get more for their money with no negative drawbacks for me, a win-win.

The combination of the popularity of kickboxing, my genuine interest in martial arts, a win-win offer, and a very repeatable process made it the perfect flame for my "Moth to Flame" protocol.

As I've mentioned many times, the strategy above is extremely repeatable, anyone can do it and you can too, and I would encourage you to.

However, if you wanted to use a different "flame", what would it be and why?

Here are some questions to consider in choosing an approach:

1. Why would people want to try this?
2. What about this makes it an easy yes?
3. Would a large number of people be interested in this?
4. Who are those people, and do they fit the avatar for the target audience for other services I offer?
5. Can I create a system around it?
6. Is that system repeatable?

7. Is this offer a win-win?

I mentioned earlier that there is only one thing that can stop you from successfully implementing the "Moth to Flame" protocol, let's talk about it.

THE CAVE YOU FEAR TO ENTER HOLDS THE TREASURE YOU SEEK!

MOTH TO FLAME

AN OFFLINE LEAD GENERATION PROTOCOL FOR NEW PERSONAL TRAINERS

THE CAVE YOU FEAR TO ENTER HOLDS THE TREASURE YOU SEEK!

The best lead generation strategy in the world will mean absolutely nothing if you cannot implement it and when it comes to the "Moth to Flame" approach, your mind will be the biggest roadblock you will face in implementing this strategy.

Have you ever heard the saying; "The cave you fear to enter holds the treasure you seek"? There are so ways you can interpret this saying. One simple way is to say that the risks and chances you fear to take, hold the opportunities you are seeking.

There is a reason most personal trainers at my gym didn't go up directly to gym members to promote their business and that reason is the fear of rejection.

Even when you have a structured approach, you will still be met with a fear to take the chance to approach a random person on the gym floor and to promote your business. Having an offer that is easy to say yes to and a structured approach makes approaching gym members many times easier than randomly striking up a conversation about their form or whatever else.

But I can promise there will be many days when you just don't feel like doing it out of fear, and that fear is keeping you out of the cave that holds your treasure (i.e., new clients, a flourishing business).

Your mind will create many excuses why it's not a good time to approach this member, why today is not a good day, and why you should just wait until... until the opportunities disappears.

Being aware of your own thoughts in these moments is important, being able to distinguish when it's actually not a good time (maybe because they are in the middle of an intense workout) vs when fear of approaching is stopping you will be a good starting point because it then allows you to change the thoughts running through your mind.

It is very important to paint a very clear picture of what you are trying to achieve and give yourself a strong and personal reason why it's important for you to achieve it, it will keep you going.

Set specific process goals.

Setting specific goals both for the number of client sessions I wanted and for the process of getting those clients was very important, however, the most important of the two is the process goal.

For me, I wanted 15 hours of personal training sessions, 3 hours per night between 5:30 pm to 8:30 pm, Monday to Friday.

When I first joined the second gym and had no clients, my process goal was:

I will be at the gym between 5:30 pm to 8:30 pm, Monday to Friday and I will approach a minimum of 10 people each day with my "Moth to Flame" offer.

Setting such a specific goal meant that I knew exactly what I needed to do each day, and it was repeatable day to day.

Pay close attention to the fact that my goal was to approach a minimum of 10 people, <u>not</u> get a minimum of 10 people to say yes.

Why is this important?

If my goal is to get a minimum of 10 people to say yes, and the first 5 people I speak to say no, I'm going to feel discouraged and may be more likely to stop approaching people.

However, if my goal is to simply approach a minimum of 10 people, that means every single approach, whether a yes or no is a success towards my goal for that day. This is more likely to keep me motivated and approaching people and I can approach 10 people every day regardless of the outcome, this is more likely to lead to success in the long run because I am more likely to stick to the plan.

As the saying goes, "The best diet is the one you can stick to consistently", the same mindset applies here.

If my goal each day is that I must get 10 gym members to say yes to my offer, if one or two days go by and in the three hours I spent at the gym in the evenings, I was unable to achieve that goal, I am more likely to feel demotivated about trying again on the third day, this can lead to me either quitting the process altogether or becoming very inconsistent.

Be clear on your "Why".

Setting a specific goal is great because you know exactly what you need to do, but you still need to do it. This is where being clear on why achieving your business and financial goals is important to you can be one of the keys to staying motivated.

Make this very personal, how will it change you or your life?

Having a strong why will give you something to pull from and use when having that pep talk with yourself in your head before approaching that one more person on the gym floor, you will be surprised how important and useful it will prove to be in helping you push forward when your mind starts looking for a reason not to enter the cave.

Find more sources of motivation.

There was one more thing that I did in the car on my drive to the gym. I played a motivational video from YouTube.

If you rolled your eyes at the idea of watching motivational videos as a way to motivate yourself to complete your mission for that day, then you are half right, but only half.

Watching motivational videos almost seem like a cheesy thing to do. However, there is a reason motivational videos on YouTube get hundreds of thousands if not millions of views. It's because they are great for getting you fired up. I know this because even before becoming a personal trainer, as someone that was always involved in sports growing up, I've always loved watching motivational videos, it gets me fired up.

One valid criticism of these videos is that they only keep you motivated in the short term, if you watch a video today, the motivation you get from it today probably won't carry over into next week.

What does work is listening to motivational videos right before you are about to take the action that you want to take. For me, that was in the car on my drive to the gym, so I was fired up as I got to the gym.

Remember "the catalyst" from my first gym? There were plenty of times when I would walk into a small storage room we had at that gym, he would be in there by himself, with his headphones on and his eyes closed with a video playing on his phone.

One day I asked him what he was doing, he mentioned that he was playing some motivational videos on YouTube and finished off his sentence by saying "They really work though, don't they". Almost as if he was surprised.

I replied, "They do!", because I had watched motivational videos for years and always felt fired up by them.

He also was playing motivational videos on his phone in that small storage him right before he would then go outside to do what he does.

When I look back on that moment, I realize that this guy (the catalyst), who on the surface initially seemed like he just had no issues walking up to gym members, approaching them, and turning them into paying clients, also had to find ways to keep himself motivated.

When I moved to the second gym and built up a client base in 9 weeks, I realized that people at that gym were looking at me the same way I looked at him (the catalyst) and would ask me questions about what I was doing and how.

They also may have been unaware that I was playing motivational videos in the car right before getting to the gym to get me fired up to do the things that I needed to do.

The point is, you should take advantage of whatever source of motivation you can find that will help you to consistently work towards your goals, whatever it is.

The specific video I played in the car was: "I CAN, I WILL, I MUST" speech by Eric Thomas featured in the first 3 minutes and 55 seconds of the video below.

This fired me up every single time and I would repeat along with the video "I CAN, I WILL, I MUST!".

Scan the QR code below for a link to the video.

Do not underestimate the importance of having the right mindset, so whether it's a motivational video or another source, you should do everything you can to get yourself in the state of mind to go after the goals you have set for yourself and the life you want for yourself.

FINAL CONSIDERATIONS

MOTH TO FLAME

AN OFFLINE LEAD GENERATION PROTOCOL FOR NEW PERSONAL TRAINERS

FINAL CONSIDERATIONS

In this section, I will briefly touch on some of the final considerations for implementing the "Moth to Flame" protocol.

We will touch on the importance of managing your expectations and how not doing so could lead to failure.

I will touch on my perspective on rejection and how it gave me more confidence to approach more people on the gym floor.

And finally, the importance of taking imperfect action.

Manage your expectations.

When I look at some of the other factors that contributed to being able to build up a client base in 9 weeks, it's important to note that the 3 years of experience I had at the previous gym was a factor.

As a new personal trainer stepping into the industry and a commercial gym for the first time, there might be other things you could stumble on that I didn't, because I had already stumbled on them in the past.

There are things you may need to learn, as well as confidence that you have to build first.

Some examples include:

1. Learning to conduct an effective consultation.

After 3 previous years as a personal trainer, I had conducted plenty of consultations and developed a style of my own, and more importantly, I had built up confidence doing so.

I didn't spend any energy wondering about how to conduct a consultation or what I should say or questions to ask.

I had done so plenty of times in the past and even already had consultation templates.

> 2. I was confident in writing programs and delivering a wide variety of sessions for different people with different needs.

This is important because it meant that I viewed everyone as a potential client because at that point, I had trained a wide variety of clients with different needs and there were no concerns in my mind about whether I had the skills to help people. I also knew that even if I didn't know something, I could do the research to find out or refer people.

You may come across a wide variety of people at the gym, some of them may have particular needs that you may not feel equipped to deal with as a new personal trainer.

There are things you have to consider if someone has a bad back, a bad knee, scoliosis and even just dealing with different personality types.

I had an underlying confidence that I could cater to a wide variety of clients and because of this I was able to focus solely on building my client base and I approached everyone.

There is a learning curve you have to go on as a new personal trainer, the qualification you completed covers only the basics and it's in the real world, with actual clients that you will learn a lot by seeing what works, doing your research when you come across a situation that you haven't before and building up your experience.

This is not to say that you should shy away from different clients with different needs, it's an opportunity to learn and improve your skill and if you really feel you cannot help someone with a particular need then you can refer them to another trainer who can.

However, as a new PT set your expectation to know that a big part of your journey at the beginning will be learning, even though you have completed your PT course.

Ultimately the confidence I had in myself, and my service due to previous years of experience is something I believe helped speed up the pace of building up my client.

These are things to keep in mind and use to set your expectations, not excuses not to push forward with the approaches.

Manage your expectations and allow for room to grow and develop confidence in yourself and your service. The more confident you become, the more it will reflect in the way you speak about your offer and speak about your service when approaching members on the gym floor.

Rejection

Speaking of setting your expectation, you should 100% expect that some people will say no, regardless of how good of a thing you are offering.

I'm willing to bet if you walked into the street and offer people £1 million in return for a high five, somebody would decline the offer.

You should expect rejection, when I say rejection, I mean people saying no to your offer. However, at the core of it, it's the fear of rejection that may stop you from going to that gym member and following the script.

As well as all the other mindset hacks that we spoke about in the previous section of the book, there is one simple hack that I used specifically around rejection that encouraged me to approach more people even with the possibility of rejection.

I simply told myself, "I'm going to give everyone the opportunity to say no to this kickboxing trial".

Any time I saw an opportunity to make an approach and the little voice in my head says:

"Ah, they look like they know what they're doing, they won't need a personal trainer."

I would respond back to that little voice with:

"That's okay, I'm going to approach them anyway and give them the opportunity to say no".

It takes anyway the pressure and allows me to make the approach and let it play out as it may.

Your mind will come up with creative reasons why you should not approach, and these mind hacks are different ways you can silence and negate those excuses. Ultimately by having that mindset, I approached more people which led to more people saying yes to the trial.

A trial does not mean a client, but the more trials (a.k.a. leads) you have the more clients you convert; it all starts with the approach.

Using this phrase worked for me mentally, it's a form of mind-hacking. In my own words, mind hacking is a way to re-structure your thoughts/perspective or view on life in a way that allows you to take action that ultimately helps you to achieve your goals.

A final note on this topic is, don't take it personal. Someone declining your offer is not personal, don't take it as such.

Take Imperfect Action

You'll do more and get more done by taking imperfect action.

The simple mindset of not feeling as though all the stars have to align before you make an approach or do whatever else you are wanting to do will allow you to go a lot further than you will if you always waited for the perfect moment.

Take imperfect action and improve as you go along.

CONCLUSION

MOTH TO FLAME

AN OFFLINE LEAD GENERATION PROTOCOL FOR NEW PERSONAL TRAINERS

CONCLUSION

Statistics say that most personal trainers fail within the first year, maybe they became a personal trainer because they love training themselves so much that they thought, "Why not make this my job". They might have seen a personal trainer with his or her client and thought, "I can do that, I train my friends all the time" They fail to approach their personal training business like a business right from the beginning.

The 80% of personal trainers that fail in the first year are not bad personal trainers, but most likely they were bad at the business of personal training, they couldn't figure it out, and it's not what they signed up for.

Becoming successful as a personal trainer will require personal growth, the type that comes from pushing yourself to go out of your comfort zone and make something happen out of nothing.

They say the harder your work the luckier you get, and you create your own luck by creating a plan of action, deciding the steps to take, and following it through.

This book is an outline of some of the steps I have taken and the protocol I have decided on after three years of trying a lot of other things and I believe you will find success with it too.

However, having a protocol, planning, and outlining the steps to get there is not enough. The secret to your success will be in the execution of the plan, not the plan itself, how consistent and disciplined you are in implementing the daily steps will determine your success.

The "Moth to Flame" protocol is the most successful offline protocol I've found in my seven-year journey so far as a personal trainer. In this book, I have outlined both the physical and mental steps I took to implement it, both the physical gym floor steps and scripts and the mental preparation are as important as each other, your mindset and state of mind is what will propel you to successfully implement the gym floor strategy.

I wish you great success as a personal trainer.

You've got this!

THE END

MOTH TO FLAME

AN OFFLINE LEAD GENERATION PROTOCOL FOR NEW PERSONAL TRAINERS

If you took anything away from this book, I would love to read your feedback and comments.

Please leave your comments and takeaways by reviewing this book on the Amazon page.

MOTH TO FLAME

AN OFFLINE LEAD GENERATION PROTOCOL FOR NEW PERSONAL TRAINERS

MOTH TO FLAME

AN OFFLINE LEAD GENERATION PROTOCOL FOR NEW PERSONAL TRAINERS